Fluid and Electrolyte

(Nursing)

TABLE OF CONTENTS

Fluids and Electrolytes: Quick Guide

Normal Range of Electrolytes Values

pH	7.35 - 7.45
$PaCO_2$	35 - 45 mmHg
HCO_3^-	22 - 26 mEg/L
Sodium	135-145 mEq/L
Potassium	3.5-5 mEq/L
Blood Urea Nitrogen (BUN)	7-20 mg/dl
Chloride	100 - 106 mEq/L
Phosphate	0.8 - 1.5 mEq/L
Magnesium	0.7 - 1.5 mEq/L
Calcium	2.2 - 2.6 mEq/L
Hematocrit (PCV)	40-50%
Urine specific gravity	1.002-1.030
Glucose	60-110 mg/dl
Osmolality	275-295

U.S.A Measurement	Metric Measurement
¼ ounce	8 grams
½ ounce	15 grams
1 ounce	30 grams
4 ounces	115 grams
8 ounces (1/2 **pound**)	225 grams
16 ounces (**1 pound**)	450 grams
32 ounces (2 **pounds**)	900 grams
35.2 ounces (2.2 **pounds**)	1 kilogram (Kg)

Volume Measurement Conversion

U.S Measurement	Metric Measurement
1 teaspoon	5 milliliters (ml)
1 tablespoon	15 mls
1 fluid ounce (2 tablespoon)	30 mls
2 fluid ounces (1/4 cup)	60 mls
8 fluid ounces (1 **cup**)	240 mls
16 fluid ounces (2 cups - **1**	480 mls
32 fluid ounces (2 cups - 1	950 mls
128 fluid ounces (4 quarts -	3.75 liters

Common Electrolytes: Causes, Signs and Symptoms

Causes of Hyponatremia
- Congestive Cardiac failure
- Nephrosis
- Cirrhosis
- Excess fluid intake
- Syndrome of Inappropriate Antidiuretic Hormone (SIADH) secretion – this causes dilutional hyponatremia
- Sodium depletion
- Loss of body fluids without replacement such as in diuretic therapy, use of laxatives, nasogastric suctioning
- Hypoaldosteronism
- Cerebral salt-wasting disease

Signs and Symptoms of Hyponatremia
- Anorexia
- Lethargy
- Dizziness
- Muscle cramp
- Muscle weakness
- Seizures
- Dry skin
- Edema

Causes of Hypernatremia
- Loss of water through GI like diarrhea or vomiting
- Loss of water from the lungs – hyperventilation
- Loss of water from the skin through Burns
- Fluid restriction
- Hypertonic IV solutions
- Tube feeding
- Hypothalamic lesions
- Cushing syndrome
- Primary hyperaldosteronism
- Diabetes insipidus (causes diuresis)

Signs and Symptoms of Hypernatremia
- Increased thirst
- Swollen tongue
- Lethargy
- Restlessness
- Weakness

Note: Replacing sodium loss rapidly can lead to a neurological disorder known as **Central Pontine Myelinolysis**, which is caused by severe damage of the myelin sheath or nerve cells in the brain stem.

Signs and Symptoms of Central pontine myelinolysis
- Sudden paralysis
- Dysphagia
- Dysarthria
- Double vision
- Loss of consciousness

Causes of Hyperkalemia

- Excess K+ intake
- Multiple blood transfusions
- Burns
- Decreased renal excretion
- Crush injuries
- Addison's disease

Signs and Symptoms of Hyperkalemia

- Muscle cramps
- Urine abnormalities
- Respiratory distress
- Reduced cardiac contractility
- Flaccid paralysis
- Irritability
- Abdominal cramps
- Abdominal distension
- Anxiety
- Dysrhythmias
- Tall tented T waves
- Absent P waves
- Prolonged PR interval and QRS duration

Signs and symptoms of Hypokalemia

- Fatigue
- Anorexia
- Decreased bowel motility
- Decreased reflexes
- Ventricular fibrillation
- Abdominal distention
- Polyuria
- Paraesthesia
- Leg cramps
- Decreased ST segment
- Prolonged PR interval
- Flat T waves

Common Causes of Hypercalcemia
- Hyperparathyroidism
- Leukaemia
- Immobilization
- Use of Diuretics

Signs and Symptoms of Hypercalcemia
- Decreased Neuromuscular excitability
- Depression of the Central Nervous System
- Constipation
- Anorexia
- Polyuria and Polydipsia
- Dehydration
- Bone pain
- Hypertension
- Short ST segment
- Bradycardia

Common Causes of Hypocalcemia

- Diarrhea
- Dietary deficiency
- Excessive use of Laxative
- Malabsorption
- Pancreatitis

Signs and Symptoms of Hypocalcemia

- Increased excitability at the Neuromuscular junction
- Muscle Cramps
- Seizures
- Numbness around mouth
- Tingling sensation
- Positive trousseau sign and chvostek's sign
- Carpopedal spasm
- Bronchospasm
- Diarrhea
- Anxiety
- Prolong QT interval

Causes of Hypermagnesemia
Prolonged use of Cathartics and antacids

Signs and Symptoms of Hypermagnesemia
- Drowsiness
- Decreased reflexes
- Respiratory depression
- Muscle weakness
- Cardiac arrhythmias
- Flushing
- Hypotension
- Hypoactive reflexes
- Diaphoresis
- Cardiac arrest
- Coma
- Prolonged PR interval
- Peaked T waves

Causes of Hypomagnesemia
- Alcoholism
- Poor nutrition
- Malabsorption

Symptoms and Signs of Hypomagnesemia
- Seizures
- Cardiac arrhythmias
- Muscle cramps
- Muscle spasms
- Tetany
- Hyperactive reflexes
- Neuromuscular irritability
- Insomnia
- Mood changes
- Anorexia
- Vomiting
- Increased tendon reflexes
- Positive trousseau's sign
- Positive chvostek's sign
- Premature ventricular contractions (PVCs)
- Flat or inverted T waves
- Widened QRS complex
- Prolonged PR interval

Causes of Hypophosphatemia
- Alcoholism
- Diarrhea
- Decreased intake
- Shift into cells
- Increased excretion
- Malabsorption
- Diabetic acidosis
- Use of diuretics
- Prolonged use of Antacids
- Dialysis

Signs and Symptoms of Hypophosphatemia (Inverse relationship with calcium)
- Malaise
- Anorexia
- Paresthesias
- Confusion
- Muscle weakness
- Decreased reflexes
- Stupor
- Impaired cardiac function
- Bone pain
- Chest pain
- Seizures
- Nystagmus
- Respiratory failure

Causes of Hyperphosphatemia
- Increased intake
- Shift from cells into serum
- Hypoparathyroid disease
- Decreased excretion
- Use of Phosphate containing enemas
- Crushing injury
- Adrenal insufficiency

Signs and Symptoms of Hyperphosphatemia
- Increased neuromuscular excitability
- Low blood calcium
- Tetany
- Tachycardia
- Anorexia
- Muscle weakness
- Hyperactive reflexes
- Calcifications in the lungs, cornea, heart and kidneys

Metabolic Acidosis

Caused by accumulation of metabolic acids or loss of bicarbonates such as:

- Chronic diarrhea
- Malnutrition
- Starvation
- Renal failure
- Diabetic Ketoacidosis (DKA)
- Trauma
- Shock
- Sepsis
- Salicylate toxicity

Signs and Symptoms of Metabolic Acidosis

- Nausea
- Headache
- Stupor
- Lethargy
- Abdominal pain
- Anorexia
- Confusion
- Coma
- Kussmaul breathing
- Vomiting
- Diarrhea

In metabolic acidosis, the body tries to compensate by increasing respiratory rate (Hyperventilation) so that the lungs excrete more CO_2

Causes of Metabolic Alkalosis

Deficit of metabolic acids or increase of bicarbonate following

- Vomiting
- NG suctioning
- Prolonged use of Antacids
- Use of diuretics

Signs and Symptoms of Metabolic Alkalosis

- Tetany
- Increased neuromuscular irritability
- Confusion
- Seizures
- Lethargy
- Coma
- Anorexia
- Paralytic ileus (due to hypokalemia)
- Dizziness
- Tremors
- Hyperreflexia
- Paraesthesia
- Muscle cramps
- Arrhythmias

Causes of Respiratory Acidosis

- Use of drugs like Narcotics and benzodiazepines that depress the respiratory system
- Decreased alveolar ventilation due to lung disease
- Impaired neuromuscular function

Signs and Symptoms of Respiratory Acidosis

- Headache
- Stupor
- Lethargy
- Tremors
- Confusion
- Seizures
- Cardiac arrhythmias
- Hypotension
- Peripheral vasodilation
- Weak thready pulse
- Warm flushed skin
- Dyspnea (difficulty in breathing)
- Slow shallow respirations
- Hypoxia and hypoventilation
- Cyanosis
- Papilledema

In respiratory acidosis, the body compensates by the kidneys retaining bicarbonates (HCO_3^-)

Causes of Respiratory Alkalosis

- Hyperventilation
- Sepsis or infection
- Hepatic cirrhosis

Signs and symptoms of Respiratory Alkalosis

- Diaphoresis
- Seizures
- Coma
- Neuromuscular irritability
- Carpopedal spasms
- Tingling in fingers and around moth
- paresthesia, dizzyness, confusion, tetany, convulsion, numb/tingling, light headed, anxiety/panic, Loss of consciousness, hyperactive reflexes

In respiratory alkalosis, the kidneys excrete more bicarbonates (HCO_3^-)

Types of Volume Expanders

Crystalloids
These types of fluids help to maintain balance between intravascular and extravascular compartments.

Examples include:
- Normal Saline   0.9% NaCl
- Hypertonic Saline   3% NaCl
- D5W (5% dextrose water)
- Lactated ringers solution – composed of NaCl, Sodium Lactate, KCl, and CaCl

Advantages of Crystalloids
- They are cheap
- Non-allergenic
- No transmission of infection
- No interference with coagulation

Disadvantages of Crystalloids
- Higher volume needed to correct fluid deficit
- Remains in the intravascular space for a short time

Colloids
These fluid types draws fluid from interstitial spaces into the intravascular compartment
Examples include:
- Dextran
- Hetastarch
- Albumin

Advantages of Colloids
- Better at expanding plasma volume than crystalloids
- May be salt sparing

Disadvantages of Colloids
- They are expensive
- Have risk of allergy in some patients
- May cause coagulopathy
- May exacerbate tissue edema

Signs and Symptoms of Cellular swelling
- Confusion
- Nausea
- Coma
- Headache
- Lethargy
- Weight gain
- Seizure
- Twitching of muscles
- Weakness

Common causes of dehydration
- Diuretic therapy
- Vomiting
- Diarrhea
- Hemorrhage
- Decreased fluid intake
- Excessive urination

Signs and Symptoms of Dehydration
- Hypotension (dizziness)
- Weak and rapid pulse
- Decreased skin turgor
- Dry mucous membranes
- Reduced tears secretion
- Reduced urine output

EXTRAs

Symptoms and Signs of intracellular dehydration

- Lethargy
- Confusion
- Coma
- Pulmonary edema
- Elevated temperature
- Seizure
- Dryness of mucous membranes
- Elevated reflexes

Signs of Hypoglycemia

- Excessive hunger
- Tachycardia
- Restlessness
- Diaphoresis
- Dizziness
- Convulsions (especially in children)

Signs of Hyperglycemia

- Excessive thirst
- Increased appetite
- Weight loss
- Blurring of vision
- Frequent urination

Cranial Nerves and functions
- CN I – Olfactory Nerve for smell
- CN II – Optic Nerve for sight
- CN III – Oculomotor nerve, moves eyes and dilates pupil
- CN IV – Trochlear nerve – moves eye
- CN V – Trigeminal nerve – for facial sensation
- CN VI – Abducens nerve – moves eye
- CN VII – Facial nerve – moves facial muscles and controls salivation
- CN VIII – Vestibulocochlear nerve for Hearing and balance
- CN IX – Glossopharyngeal nerve for taste and swallow
- CN X – Vagus nerve – controls heart rate and digestion
- CN XI – Spinal Accessory nerve – controls muscles that move the head
- CN XII – Hypoglossal nerve – moves the tongue

Left sided Heart failure

- Fatigue
- Tachypnea
- Cough
- Orthopnea (difficulty in breathing upon lying down)
- Restlessness
- Cyanosis (bluish discoloration)
- Extreme weakness
- Dyspnea (Difficulty in breathing)

Right sided Heart failure

- Distended neck veins
- Edema of the legs
- Ascites
- Hepatomegaly
- Oliguria
- Anorexia
- Cyanosis
- Bloating

ENTERAL ROUTES: Oral, Sublingual, Rectal and Buccal

Benefits: Convenient to take and good absorption

Disadvantages: cannot be used for unconscious patients, first pass effect reduces the availability of drug and can cause irritation of mucosal lining

PARENTERAL ROUTES: Intradermal, Subcutaneous, Intravenous, Intrathecal, Intramuscular, Intramedullary, Intraperitoneal, Intra-articular and Intra-arterial.

Benefits: very rapid or immediate onset and drug can still be administered even to an unconscious patient

Disadvantages: aseptic procedure required, expensive and risk of injury to nerves

INHALATIONAL ROUTES: Nose or Mouth

Benefit: rapid onset with large area for absorption of drug

Disadvantage: dosage of drug absorbed cannot be regulated

TOPICAL ROUTES: Skin, Nose, Ear, and Eye

Benefit: drug acts where needed without systemic effect

Disadvantages: slow onset; it can cause local reaction and applicable to few drugs

Levels of Consciousness

- **Fully Conscious:** completely awake and alert
- **Confusion:** continuous disorientation, forgetfulness, difficulty following commands and agitation
- **Lethargy:** Alert and oriented in time, place and person; sleeps frequently but can awake to voice or tapping
- **Obtundation:** extremely drowsy with little responsiveness and needs vigorous simulation to awaken; stays awake for some seconds and sleeps again.
- **Stupor:** minimal movement with little response to stimuli by groaning or moaning and only awakes when repeatedly stimulated.
- **Coma:** lack of response to stimuli even to pain

Drug overdose/Poisons and their Antidotes

Drug/Poison	Antidote
Anticholinesterase	Atropine
Acetaminophen	N-acetylcysteine (Mucomyst)
Anticholinergic agent	Physostigmine
Anticoagulants	Vitamin K or Protamine or Fresh Frozen Plasma
Benzodiazepines	Flumazenil (romazicon)
Cyclophosphamide	Mesna
Beta blockers	Glucagon or Insulin
Calcium channel blockers	Glucagon or Insulin
Digoxin, Digitoxin	Digoxin immune Fab (digibind)
Isoniazid	Pyridoxine
Methotrexate	Leucovorin calcium
Warfarin	Phytonadione (Vitmin K)
Tricyclic antidepressant	Sodium bicarbonate or physostigmine
Heparin	Protamine sulphate
Doxorubicin	Dexrazoxane
Opiates	Naloxone (narcan) or Nalmefene (revex)
Iron	Deferoxamine
Flourouracil	Leucovorin calcium
Sulfonylurea	Octreotide or Glucose

Drug overdose/Poisons and their Antidotes

Drug/Poison	Antidote
Aspirin	Sodium bicarbonate
Carbon monoxide	Oxygen
Cyanide	Hydroxycobalamin, Amyl nitrite or Sodium Thiosulfate
Insulin	Glucose
Alcohol withdrawal	Librium
Arsenic	Dimercaprol
Lead	EDTA or Succimer (DMSA)
Copper	Penicillamine
Mercury	Succimer (DMSA)
Hydrofluoric acid	Calcium gluconate
Ethylene glycol	Fomepizole or Ethanol
Serotonin reuptake inhibitors	Cyproheptadine
Methemoglobin	Methylene blue

Positioning of Patients

- **Fowlers Position:** a position where the trunk and head are raised to 40- 90 degrees while the lower limbs lie on the bed. This position is used for patients with breathing problems, those with NG tubes and cardiac disorders.
- **Cardiac Position**: when the head and trunk of the patient is raised to the 45 degrees. Used is patients with cardiac disorders.
- **Lithotomy Position:** In this position, the patient lies with the back while the legs are raised to hip level or above the hip and often supported with stirrups. It is used during delivery or gynecological procedures
- **Sim's Position:** in this, the patient lies on the side with the hip joint flexed so that the knee approaches the chest. The upper arm is flexed at the elbow. This is used in perineal examinations such as digital rectal examination or when examining the prostate or in upper GI endoscopy. Pregnant women feel more comfortable lying for long in this position.
- **Trendelenburg Position:** in this, the patient lies flat on a couch while the head of the bed is lowered further so that the legs are higher than the level of the head. This is used in hernia surgeries and in setting central line.
- **Reverse Trendelenburg Position:** the patient lies flat while the bed is inclined such that the head is higher than the level of the legs. It prevents aspiration during surgeries and in patients at risk of aspiration.

- **Supine Position**: Lying flat with the back on the bed. The commonly used position for most surgeries and for examination of patients.
- **Prone Position:** lying flat with the stomach touching the bed while the face is turned to the side. Used for back surgeries.
- **Lateral position:** lying on your side with the upper arm flex. This could be **left lateral** when the left side touches the bed or **right lateral position** when the right side touches the bed.

Types of Insulin

Type of Insulin	Onset	Peak	Duration
RAPID ACTING			
Insulin Lispro	15 – 30 min	30min to 2hr 30min	3 – 6 hr
Insulin Aspart	10 – 20 min	1 – 3 hr	3 – 5 hr
Insulin Glulisine	10 – 15 min	1 to 1hr 30min	3 – 5 hr
SHORT ACTING			
Regular Insulin	30 – 60 min	1 – 5 hr	6 – 10 hr
INTERMEDIATE ACTING			
NPH Insulin	1 – 2 hr	6 – 14 hr	16 – 24 hr
LONG ACTING			
Insulin glargine	70 min	None	18 – 24 hr
Insulin detemir	1 – 2 hr	12 – 24 hr	Varies

Glasgow Coma Scale

A scale use to assess the level of consciousness following traumatic brain injury. A score of 8 or less is severe brain injury; A score of 9 – 12 is moderate brain injury; A score of 13 – 15 is mild brain injury

Eye Opening (E)
- 4 - spontaneous
- 3 - to sound
- 2 - to pressure
- 1 - none
- NT - not testable

Verbal Response (V)
- 5 - orientated
- 4 - confused
- 3 - utter incoherent words
- 2 – utter sounds, but no words
- 1 - none
- NT - not testable

Motor Response (M)
- 6 - obeys command
- 5 - localizing
- 4 - normal flexion
- 3 - abnormal flexion
- 2 - extension
- 1 - none
- NT - not testable

APGAR SCORE

This is a score used to check a baby's health immediately after delivery

PARAMETER	SCORE 0	SCORE 1	SCORE 2
Appearance	Generalized bluish discoloration	Bluish color at the extremities	No blue color
Pulse	No pulse	Pulse < 100 beats/min	Pulse > 100 beats/min
Grimace	No response to stimulation	Grimace or feeble cry when stimulated	Sneezing or coughing or pulling away when stimulated
Activity	No movement	Some movement	Active movement
Respiration	No breathing	Weak, slow or irregular breathing	Strong and regular breathing

Apgar Score of 7 and above are generally normal, 4 to 6 fairly low, and 3 and below are generally regarded as critically low.